YOU TOO CAN SURVIVE

YOU TOO CAN SURVIVE

◆

My Journey as an Alzheimer's Caregiver

Jean Pitzer

iUniverse, Inc.
New York Lincoln Shanghai

YOU TOO CAN SURVIVE
My Journey as an Alzheimer's Caregiver

iUniverse books may be ordered through booksellers or by contacting:

iUniverse
2021 Pine Lake Road, Suite 100
Lincoln, NE 68512
www.iuniverse.com
1-800-Authors (1-800-288-4677)

The views expressed in this work are solely those of the author and do not necessarily reflect the views of the publisher, and the publisher hereby disclaims any responsibility for them.

ISBN: 978-0-595-41068-2 (pbk)
ISBN: 978-0-595-85428-8 (ebk)

Printed in the United States of America

To the memory of Gordon

and

To my children for their love and support

Contents

Acknowledgments ix

Introduction xi

CHAPTER 1   Early Signs 1

CHAPTER 2   Accepting the Situation 4

CHAPTER 3   Support from Friends 7

CHAPTER 4   Taking the Keys Away 9

CHAPTER 5   Day Care 11

CHAPTER 6   Sometimes Loved Ones Don't Understand 15

CHAPTER 7   Support from Our Church, Family, and Friends 17

CHAPTER 8   Labeling Objects and Other Stories 20

CHAPTER 9   Stories That Will Make You Cry 25

CHAPTER 10   Stories to Amuse You 28

CHAPTER 11   Once in a While, We Get It Right 30

CHAPTER 12   Looking for a Nursing Home 34

CHAPTER 13   The Last Few Days 38

CHAPTER 14   Helpful Suggestions 45

CHAPTER 15   Conclusion 47

You Too Can Survive 49

Acknowledgments

John Pitzer for encouraging me to do this book

Joyce Peden for editing

Molly Pitzer for the book cover

Shannon Pitzer for computer help

Jim Pitzer

Lynne and Bruce Anderson

Tommy Peden

Joe and Mary Lou Gay

Rosemary and the late Jimmy Duncan

Jean King

Mary Jo and the late Dick Patten

Bill Cobb

Bob and Ruth Juhler

A. D. Draughn

Vern and Jean Daugherty

Norbert Lodygowski

Rev. Mr. Alan Farquhar

Jerry McCurdy

Rhonda Talamo

Susan Ashley

The Westminster Church family

The volunteers of the Medical Center of Arlington

The Bridge Group

Introduction

I have been urged by several friends to write about my experiences dealing with my husband's Alzheimer's. It's not that I have all the answers, but if any of my experiences or suggestions can help a single person living the life of a caregiver, then I am thrilled. My focus is on day-to-day activities and how we tried to get through life one day at a time.

I first heard about Alzheimer's disease around 1985. I thought at first that a new illness had been identified. Upon further investigation, I learned that the disease had been known before as senility, hardening of the arteries, or dementia. Dr. Alzheimer was a German physician who died in 1915, so we were rather slow in getting the correct diagnosis for this disease that eventually destroys the brain.

Gordon and I met at Sterling College, a small Presbyterian school in Sterling, Kansas. He was just home from World War II and was anxious to get on with his life. He had come to Sterling from Pennsylvania. I was a sophomore from Oklahoma when we met. We had both lived through the Depression and World War II.

We married after I finished my sophomore year, and I went to work in order for my husband to get an education. That probably seems foolish to today's young people, but it was expected of young wives in 1947.

We eventually ended up living in Texas and had two wonderful sons, Jim and John. Both of the boys graduated from Sterling like their father did, and Jim met his wife there—again like his father. Jim married Shannon in 1979, and they had two beautiful daughters, Jessica and Molly, born in 1982 and 1983 respectively.

Our other son, John, became a priest in the Catholic Church. Gordon's buttons popped off with pride as each son made his way in life. They both shared Gordon's huge interest in sports, and it was something that gave them many enjoyable hours together. But with our little granddaughters, Gordon had a very special relationship and the girls were delighted that Grandpa was their grandfather.

After Gordon retired, he was thrilled to be able to babysit the girls when Shannon had other things to do. Shannon did not work away from home at the time but was very involved with church work and other things that often required a babysitter. He enjoyed taking them to the park to play. They would sometimes go to a movie or play games at home. The three of them had a strong, special bond.

As the girls grew, they became more active in extracurricular activities. We always went to the games, concerts, and plays they were involved in.

When Gordon became ill the girls were sad, but more than anything, they were frightened. They didn't know what was happening to Grandpa. He was still happy to see them, but things were different. He didn't always remember to ask about their school activities, their dates, or their friends.

Since Gordon's death, both girls have graduated from high school and now they attend college. He wanted so much to witness these things but was unable to. He wasn't here to find out that Jessica is engaged to be married. He wasn't here to see Molly go to Northern Ireland as a missionary with the Youth for Christ organization. I know he would have been so proud to see his beautiful granddaughters blossom into adulthood. But it was not to be.

1

Early Signs

My husband had always been an exceptionally healthy person. As a young man he seldom went to a doctor. As an adult, it became a source of pride for him. However, in 1995, at the age of seventy-one, after several visits to a urologist, he was told that he had prostate cancer. He had a look of disbelief on his face when he arrived home to tell me about it. He had the necessary surgery and spent a couple of days in the hospital. This was his first time in a hospital as a patient since 1950, when he had a ruptured appendix.

Within a month after his surgery, I realized that something was wrong. He was confused, forgetful, and things were just "not right." I questioned a friend who had had the same surgery a year earlier, and he had none of the symptoms Gordon was having. Later I learned of other, similar stories in which there seemed to be some kind of connection between anesthesia and dementia.

One of the first things I noticed was a change in his personality. Gordon had always been a quiet, passive person. Now, if something happened that he didn't like, he started to yell at me. This was something he had never done in our more than forty years of marriage. One night he was driving home and another couple was in the car with us. We entered an area of town that had different speed zones prominently posted and a strict law enforcement crew to deal with those who didn't adhere. We needed to slow down from forty to thirty-five MPH. When Gordon made no attempt to slow down, I suggested he do so.

To my surprise, he yelled, "But I'm only going forty-five!" After a couple of other instances like this, I knew for sure that something was wrong.

Gordon was due to have his annual physical shortly after this time. When I asked if he wanted me to go with him, he gave me a definite no. I decided then to write a letter to our family doctor to tell him that Gordon was coming in, and I listed the concerns I had. I made an appointment for myself a few days later to talk to the doctor about Gordon. The doctor was shocked to find Gordon in such a condition and told us to see a neurologist. I told the doctor that if Gordon learned he had Alzheimer's, he would just give up and not try to fight it. The doctor, though, firmly believed in every patient knowing his or her own condition. Thus, the tests began.

Gordon was not happy about the tests he had to go through, but he did what the doctor told him he must do. First, he was given a blood test to see if he had ever had Lyme disease. Gordon's symptoms could have been the result of Lyme even from a blood transfusion. Next was an MRI to check for a brain tumor, and then an EEG to check brain wave malfunctions. All of the tests were negative, and the doctor said we could assume it was Alzheimer's.

Sitting in the doctor's office after that, it felt like I had been hit by a truck. In some ways, I had been expecting the doctor to tell us exactly what he did. But I knew that our world would never be the same. I'm not really sure if you can ever be prepared for this kind of news. Moving forward was the only option for us at this point.

After the doctor gave us this dreaded news, we walked twenty feet to the car. Gordon attempted to differentiate between his friend's illness and his own.

"Ken has Alzheimer's, and I have Parkinson's."

I told him, "You have it backward. Ken has Parkinson's, and you have Alzheimer's."

I got just about as much response from him as if I'd commented on the weather.

I immediately called both of our sons and also Gordon's family in Pennsylvania to tell them the news. They were all very supportive and offered to help in any way possible, but I knew that I would be the day-to-day caregiver, and I was very frightened for him and for myself. I had never had close contact with an Alzheimer's patient, and I didn't have any confidence that I could help Gordon, let alone do it right. I had heard stories of how the patients become unable to care for themselves. The disease robs them of their ability to dress and bathe or attend to themselves in the bathroom. I had also heard that they have a tendency to get lost or run away.

At the drugstore, I found a video that had been put out by Dr. C. Everett Koop, Surgeon General of the United States at the time. Dr. Koop had videos on several different diseases, and I found the one on Alzheimer's to be very helpful. I saw from the video what to expect from the disease and what to expect from the patient. I learned that some doctors think 25–50 percent of the children of Alzheimer's patients will inherit the disease. Those statistics have been disputed by some, but they are still very frightening.

After I watched the video a couple of times, I had my sons and my daughter-in-law watch it. Then I sent the tape to Gordon's brother and sister. This was not to frighten them but to help them understand what to expect from Gordon and how they could better understand the situation and help care for him when we were all together.

2

Accepting the Situation

After getting over the initial shock of the diagnosis, we attempted, as best we could, to resume a normal life. Things remained much the same for months. We both continued to volunteer at the Medical Center of Arlington two afternoons a week. Gordon still enjoyed his yard work, and we were both active in our Presbyterian church ...

Life went on.

When we got up in the mornings, things were usually pretty good. Early morning is the best time of day for someone with this disease. As the hours passed, he would become more confused about what we were doing and why. This is a common occurrence with Alzheimer's patients. It is called "sun downing."

Gordon enjoyed watching TV, and he always read *Sports Illustrated* and the sports page of the newspaper. When he tired of that, he would work for a while in the yard, but he quickly lost the strength to push the lawn mower.

He continued to have a good appetite and wanted to feed himself although he often missed his mouth. I was able to find long plastic adult bibs to protect his clothes, and I bought two of them so he would not be embarrassed by my not having one.

Gradually things changed. He needed more help in dressing. I had to start helping him shower and shave. By now he had to wear pads that were very much like diapers. He never seemed to be able to get them on without my help. He had many questions about why he could not handle these tasks alone. I tried to convince him that he would soon feel better and would be able to do all these things by himself.

The most difficult time for me was when Gordon got frustrated because he couldn't remember a name or a word. He would pound his fist on the arm of his recliner and ask over and over, "Why can't I remember?"

This was new territory for both of us, and I didn't know how to answer him. I would tell him it was the disease kicking in. It seemed to help him calm down. Then I realized the doctor was right in insisting that all patients know their own diagnosis. Some Alzheimer's patients have no clue as to what is wrong with them, and I think that can only complicate matters. They know things are not normal, but they have no clue as to why.

The first medicine given to Gordon was Cognex. It helped clear his mind, and the thought process was a little better, but it did not help as much as the doctor had hoped. However, it was the only medication for Alzheimer's available in 1996. There were so many potential side effects that we had to go to the lab every week to have his blood checked to see if the medicine was affecting his liver. After a couple of months we were told to come every three weeks. Finally, the new Alzheimer's drug Aricept was put on the market, and the doctor started Gordon on it right away. After six months, I could see great improvement in Gordon's speech, thought process, and ability to care for himself. This only helped for about four years, and there was no new medicine available.

Our activities outside the house were starting to be curtailed, but we still had friends who would call and invite us to a movie on Sunday afternoon. I know Gordon did not get anything out of the story line, but he would sit very quietly or, more often, would go to sleep. No one thought anything about it, and I was able to enjoy myself and know that he was all right.

3

Support from Friends

One Sunday after church, a few months after the diagnosis, a good friend came to me and asked if I had plans for the following Wednesday evening. I assured her I did not, and she proceeded to ask if I would like to go out to dinner. My first concern was Gordon, of course, but she said that her husband would come over and take Gordon out to eat as well. I accepted and had a great evening with a wonderful friend. The next Sunday, the same friend asked again if I had plans for Wednesday. Soon another friend joined us, and her husband would go with the other two men to eat. Before long, we invited two more friends who had recently been widowed, and the party grew. To this day the women still go out to dinner almost every Wednesday. We have become very close. What started out as a ministry for me has developed into a ministry for many.

After several months, the men decided they could no longer take Gordon out. He was not steady on his feet, and they were afraid of him falling, so instead they offered to bring food to the house. I was grateful but told them that if they would continue to do this every week, I would prepare dinner for them before I left with the girls. In order to make things easier for me the men would occasionally call to tell me not to cook because they were bringing hamburgers to the house. This continued until Gordon finally had to go into an assisted-living facility.

This is an example of what someone can do to help a caregiver. Take lunch or dinner over to the house. If the patient has someone to sit with them, take the caregiver out to lunch. Offer to stay with the patient while the caregiver goes to a movie or out to shop or just to a park to sit. The caregiver may even want to do something as simple as take a nap. The least little thing is appreciated more than you can imagine.

4

Taking the Keys Away

During World War II, Gordon was a jeep driver for a captain in the Army. He had a great sense of direction and was doing something he truly loved. He was happy not to be fighting on the front line of battle, and he loved driving. He told me, years later, that he got his first stripe because he was able to find his way back to camp when he and the captain got lost in France.

Before Gordon's illness, we used to go for a drive on Sunday afternoons. We drove around new neighborhoods; sometimes we drove out into the country. But as long as Gordon was behind the wheel of a car, he was perfectly happy.

Every summer we drove all the way from Texas to Pennsylvania to visit Gordon's family. One reason for this was because we both enjoyed driving, and we also could not afford to fly. I felt I owed it to Gordon's mother to go there every summer so she could spend time with her two grandsons. We also loved going to visit his friends and relatives and to leave the Texas heat for two weeks.

In 1997, a couple of years into Gordon's illness, we were listening to Paul Harvey one day when he stated that the Alzheimer's Association had announced that anyone who had been diagnosed with Alzheimer's should not be driving a car.

Gordon looked at me and said, "But I have never had any trouble driving."

I agreed with him but said, "If you should happen to have an accident while driving, the other person might try to sue us for everything we have if they found out you're an Alzheimer's patient."

He never drove again but delighted in telling people that his wife wouldn't let him drive. It certainly was not the only time I had to play the role of "bad guy," but it was something I thought had to be done.

One of Gordon's funny habits was jiggling his keys in his pocket. I knew I could not hide keys from him and was somewhat concerned that he might take my keys and try to drive. I took the car key off his key ring and put another key on it. It gave him such satisfaction to be able to carry his keys, and it comforted me to know that he would not be able to start the car.

It frightens me terribly to hear of Alzheimer's patients driving alone. Not only can they get lost, but there is a very real possibility that they might forget speed limits, to stop at red lights, or which side of the road to drive on. They also could step on the gas instead of the brake. All of these scenarios could possibly kill someone. What family could live with such a possibility? Until you have watched these patients deteriorate before your eyes, you really have no idea what they are capable of doing.

5

Day Care

With everything that was going on, I kept reading all I could about Alzheimer's disease. Reading, though, was not keeping my head above water. Being the primary caregiver was taking its toll on my health. If I continued down this path, both Gordon and I would suffer even more. I finally realized one day that I had a real problem with either depression or exhaustion—or both. I wanted to sleep all the time. I was blue and felt very tired and sad. Stress can rob you of all your strength, and I was very stressed.

More telling signs appeared as Gordon's condition worsened. As volunteers at the hospital, we are known as "runners." We stay in the runner room until there is a call. After the call comes in, we might do any number of things: discharge a patient, pick up samples for the lab, deliver mail or flowers, or escort people to different areas of the hospital. The exercise was good for both of us, and Gordon enjoyed being with his friends. Though he began having more trouble, he could still push the luggage cart while someone else took a wheelchair to discharge a patient.

While volunteering at the hospital, one of his favorite things to do was escort people to Radiology; he would insist on taking all of the calls for Radiology if he was in the room at the time.

Even the girls in Registration would come to the door and say, "Gordon, I have someone for you to take to Radiology."

They knew he felt useful when he was able to do this. One day, when asked to take someone to Radiology, he looked at me with a blank stare and said, "I don't remember where it is." That nearly broke my heart!

One day, two different volunteers came to me at the hospital to say, "Don't let Gordon go anywhere alone today."

I was already aware that he was not having a good day, but the people we worked with were so wonderful to help me watch him. That afternoon, one man caught Gordon trying to go out the front door, and later another man caught him going out the back door. He always enjoyed just standing outside looking around, and I think that was what he was doing. I realized, though, that these men were so concerned about his safety, I had no choice but to make some changes.

I decided to try an adult day care center for Gordon. It was run by the most caring group of people. They were open from 7:30 AM to 5:30 PM five days a week. I knew I could handle nights and weekends if I could just have help on weekdays.

At first Gordon spent a couple of days a week at the center, and this evolved into a five-day-a-week routine. I considered giving up my volunteer work, because I didn't want to pay thirty-five dollars a day to have my husband taken care of just so I could volunteer. Then I realized that he was going to be at day care regardless of what I was doing. In certain situations, things don't always come out black and white. There is a lot of rationalizing along the way. Things I thought I could never do soon became ordinary.

For those who will be looking for a day care center, I urge you to visit the facility when they aren't expecting you. Don't call and make an appointment. I am saying this because it is very important for you to feel comfortable with the facility. Just drop in, and then you will be sure you are getting a true picture. I found one day care center that had only straight chairs for the patients to sit in all day; that is difficult for people whose main function is to sit. The one I found, Mission Arlington Day Care, had ten or fifteen recliners, a couple of overstuffed chairs, and couches. They also had round tables (no sharp corners) for the patients to eat breakfast, lunch, and their mid-morning and afternoon snacks. Lunch was provided by Meals on Wheels. Thus, the workers did not have to divide their attention between the patients and food preparation.

Some type of craft was provided each day. Projects could be simple as stamping a house or some other object on construction paper. Then the patients were instructed to color the pictures.

They had volunteers who came in almost daily to play the piano, sing, or read to the patients. They encouraged the patients to sing along with old familiar songs. I'm sure that many did not understand the words or what was going on. But the long-term memory is the last to go, and once in a while they would remember the words from earlier days.

It became part of Gordon's routine and a break for me. There were approximately twenty patients that came most of the time, though not all of them had Alzheimer's. Some were stroke patients, and many were adults who were not able to stay alone all day while the family worked. The center had a washer and dryer and extra clothes in case of an accident. Once in a while this was a real blessing.

It had been suggested to me early in the illness that I would probably benefit from being in a support group. I contacted the Alzheimer's Association in Fort Worth, and they mailed me a list of support groups in the county. I went to one and got absolutely no help from it. There were only two people there besides myself and the leader. The two were children of Alzheimer's patients, and they had a different agenda, because neither of them were full-time caregivers, so I felt no connection with them.

Much later, I met a woman whose husband was in the day care center with Gordon. She invited me to go with her to another support group. I did and was so thankful for the invitation. There were ten or twelve ladies talking about the same things I had been going through. They discussed the difficulty of having to help get the patient out of bed or out of a chair. They struggled to get them dressed and then to keep them dressed. They stressed how tired they were because they could not get a full night's sleep, and naps were out of the question. I identified with their dilemmas immediately. Some of them had little support from family or friends, but, thankfully, I did. I continued going to this group until after Gordon went into the nursing home.

6

Sometimes Loved Ones Don't Understand

I am going to tell a story that in no way is intended to be critical of someone on the outside of this illness.

My only sister lived in Dallas, and we talked on the phone at least once a day. I had told her what was happening with Gordon and some of the things he was doing. At one point she told me that I should not be going out to dinner every week with the girls. She thought I should stay at home and take care of my husband. After all, I went to choir practice every week, and I went to my investment club meeting once a month, and that should be enough. I was very disappointed with her statement, but I let it drop, because I didn't have the energy to argue.

A couple of weeks later, our youngest son was home and called my sister. She reiterated what she said to me about staying home.

John's only answer was, "Aunt Lucille, we are not going to argue about this, but you are dead wrong."

For years I had been able to earn a little extra money by helping to proctor family practice medical examinations in Dallas. When I was still working full time, I would take a day of vacation to proctor one test a year. After I had retired, and about three years into Gordon's illness, I was asked to proctor a two-day examination. I asked my sister if she would keep Gordon one of the days. I offered to pay her the same amount I paid the day care center. She insisted that she would keep him both days.

At the end of the first day, I had just gotten home with Gordon when my sister called. She had not wanted to talk in front of Gordon so she waited until we could talk on the phone.

"There has to be some changes made," she said.

I really did not understand what she was talking about. Then she continued.

"Jean, I don't know how you do it. You must get him into a nursing home. You cannot keep him at home any longer."

I am telling this story so others will not assume to know what is going on in the life of a caregiver. If you know someone who is caring for a loved one, I urge you to call them and do something to lighten their load.

7

Support from Our Church, Family, and Friends

When friends first heard about the illness, some didn't know what to say or do. That is not unusual when dealing with Alzheimer's. However, most of our friends helped in one way or another.

I received a letter one day from our minister. He was aware that some of the members of our church were helping me, but he wanted to encourage others from the church to do their part. So, he gave me a list of four retired men who would be willing to come to the house during the day to stay with Gordon. That allowed me to go shopping, go to a movie, or do whatever I wanted and needed to do without needing to put him in adult day care. Our minister also listed four couples that were willing to help out: each husband offered to stay with Gordon so the wife and I could go out to dinner. This was in addition to the Wednesday dinner group. It might seem like a small thing, but it worked wonders for me. I tried not to abuse the privilege, but just to know that I could call on someone to help me was a wonderful feeling.

Life can change so quickly when we are faced with some type of serious illness. I sing in the choir at church and would leave Sunday school about fifteen minutes early to get to the choir room to robe and to rehearse. We have a very small church and a very small Sunday school class, so everyone was aware of what was going on.

When I was ready to leave Sunday school for choir, I would tell Gordon to remain seated with our friends and that I would see him in church. For a while, this worked well, but sometimes as soon as I left the room, Gordon would get up to follow me.

Our teacher would say, "No, Gordon, stay here with us."

He would sit for a minute and then the teacher would again have to ask him to stay in the room.

I didn't know about this for quite some time. Friends tried to shield things from me as much as possible.

As soon as Sunday school would end, another friend would take Gordon to the sanctuary and sit with him during church. If he was not going to be there, he would call me so I could arrange for someone else to sit with Gordon. Not only were these people trying to help Gordon, but they were also helping me. Having that hour on Sunday morning to relax and not have full responsibility was a godsend. I know there are cases in which the caregiver has absolutely no help from anyone. This is a very frustrating feeling, and many caregivers can feel overwhelmed. The important thing to remember is not to give up. Continue looking for help and asking questions. I am just so grateful for all the support I had.

Our Sunday school teacher, knowing how much Gordon enjoyed sports, would get tickets for just the two of them to go to a college game or to a Texas Ranger baseball game. If Gordon got tired before the game was over, they would just come home early.

Not only did he still enjoy sports, but he also enjoyed country music. In 1998, I purchased tickets to one of his favorite musical groups, the Statler Brothers. After buying the tickets, I made the mistake of telling Gordon we were going, and all day long he badgered me with questions: "What time is the show, who is going, how do we get there, what time does it start?"

Then he would start all over again. This was a definite misjudgment on my part.

Another church member, on hearing about a tutoring service for a nearby grade school, had a good idea. The church was attempting to get the retired members of the congregation involved. So this one friend thought the best way to help the tutoring program was for him to sit with Gordon, so I could get out of the house and help tutor.

Another example of assistance was my involvement with a women's investment club that meets once a month. In order for me to attend, a friend would stay with Gordon while his wife and I went to the club meeting.

The final example in this chapter has to do with a group of people that Gordon and I had been involved with for over thirty years. There were six couples that loved to play bridge, and we usually met on the first Saturday of each month for dinner and cards. When Gordon got sick, we continued to play bridge. If he needed help, one of the "dummies" of the game would stand by him to make sure he played correctly. This went on for about three years. It finally came to a point where he could no longer hold his cards and couldn't play without someone being with him constantly. I finally realized that it was time to quit the club, but they insisted we still get together just for dinner and not to play bridge. Five years later, nothing has changed except Gordon is no longer with us.

There are some serious bridge players in this group, and for them to give up playing in order not to hurt a friendship is incredible. We get so involved in our daily lives that we sometimes forget to look around and see how many kind, thoughtful, loving people there are in this world.

I honestly don't think I could have made it through this without the unbelievable support from family and friends.

8

Labeling Objects and Other Stories

I realized, about five years into the disease, that it was time to put labels on all of the appliances in the kitchen. If I asked Gordon to get something from the refrigerator, he would likely go to the microwave. The labels seemed to help, because he could still manage to read a little. Having him help me in the kitchen made him feel better about a frustrating situation. This was very important, because as stated earlier, after diagnosis, it is so easy for a patient to sit and do nothing.

When friends came to the house and saw the labels on all of the appliances, it was probably the first time some of them realized how bad things had become.

One day, a friend from the dinner group called to invite me to go with her and another friend to New York City for the weekend. My friend worked for an airline company and had a pass for me. I told her it depended on whether or not our son Jim could stay with his dad. When I called Jim, he not only agreed, but insisted on coming to the house to stay with his dad over the weekend.

We flew off to the Big Apple—what a fun break and what great friends! We took in a couple of Broadway shows and just had a good time. I came back rested and energized.

We returned about noon on Sunday. Jim had taken his dad to his home to eat lunch, and they returned to our house after I called to say I was home.

When they came through the door, Jim said, "See, Dad, I told you she was home."

Later he said to me, "Mother, I had no idea what you were dealing with."

At this point in the journey with Alzheimer's, I finally realized that Gordon was getting up at night without my hearing him. Every morning the house was redecorated. Knickknacks that belonged in the living room would be in the den. Things from the den would be in the kitchen. He never broke anything, but he was very busy for a couple of hours during the night.

We have two doors leading into our bedroom, and I was concerned about how to keep Gordon from wandering in the house without putting bolts on the doors. I finally came up with the idea of bells. I bought two cow bells at the hardware store. Each was approximately two inches long. I tied a string to each bell and hung them from the ceiling about two inches in front of each door. The strings were long enough so that the bells hung a couple of inches below the top of the doors. Every night when I went to bed, I "set" the bells when I closed the doors, and I was always awakened by the sound of the bells when Gordon walked out of the room.

The bells were a nonissue with him. There was no reaction at all when I set the bells, but it made me feel more secure to know that he was not up and about, possibly going outside while I slept.

One night when he got up, he flipped on the overhead light, which woke me up. I didn't say anything for a while but just watched him. He took the top sheet off our bed and put it on the toilet. I was hopeful the lid was down. Later he very carefully spread it on top of the bed again.

He then began to rearrange everything on the countertop in the bath-room. I could hear the clinking of the drinking glass, the soap dish, etc. As he started down the hall, I asked him to come back to bed.

He gave me an emphatic, "No!"

When I asked why, his only answer was, "I'm not through."

So I sat up in bed, turned on the TV, and let him go. He was extremely agitated, and I knew he had to work through it. He finally sat down on the bed for a minute, got up and did something else, and came back. After about an hour and a half, he settled down and went to sleep.

The confusion with clothing was one of the more difficult aspects to deal with. While visiting our youngest son, we went to church. When we got there, I was shocked to see that Gordon was wearing a beautiful blue plaid shirt under his navy sport coat—and under that shirt was a brown plaid shirt he had slept in the night before, when I hadn't been able to convince him to put his pajamas on. I didn't mention it to Gor-don. I don't think anyone noticed the double shirts, but if they did, most of the parishioners knew about his condition and would under-stand.

I'm sure some of you are wondering why I didn't observe him more closely. I found that he still wanted his independence. He did not want to be treated as a child. He could dress himself, and for a long time he did a good job with it. Gordon had always been very careful about his appearance, but after the illness took hold, I don't think he cared about what—if anything—he was wearing.

I also found out very quickly not to cross Gordon. If he said some-thing that was not true, I would let it pass. If I corrected him, he became angry and very agitated. It was easier to let the statement slide, and if something like that happened while we were with friends, I would discreetly frown or shake my head at them to indicate that they should not correct him, either. I found it much easier just to never contradict him, and our friends certainly understood.

One trait of Alzheimer's can be very aggressive behavior. There were times when he became very belligerent, and I didn't think it wise to question him about it. This seems to vary with different patients. Gordon had never been an aggressive person, so he didn't get angry very often. But when he did, it was frightening. Some patients actually get violent with a loved one during these times. I am so thankful that I did not have to experience that. If you do experience violent behavior with the person you are caring for, I would suggest you call for help immediately.

There was a period of time when Gordon would walk out of the bedroom with absolutely nothing on. At one point his family was visiting from Pennsylvania. I told them that I would try to watch Gordon very carefully but not to be shocked if he appeared without his clothes. One day, he was in the bathroom. I decided I should check on him and met him in the hallway coming toward the den. He was naked. Luckily, I was the only one to see him, but this is one of the things you have to watch for with an Alzheimer's patient.

One morning, Gordon got up feeling good, and the day looked hopeful. But within an hour, he was talking incoherently nonstop. I tried to make sense out of it, but there was no way I could. Every time his eyes landed on something, he added that object to what he was saying. He finally started talking about children and made it very clear that he needed to talk to someone with children. I asked if he wanted to talk to Jim or Shannon, so I called their home. Shannon answered. I told her that Dad needed to talk to someone with children, and she agreed to talk to him. He talked for ten minutes, completely incoherently. For example, he saw an envelope—a piece of junk mail—and he picked it up.

"I have a letter from Jean's mother," he said, referring to the junk mail. (My mother had been dead for about six years at that time.)

After the conversation finally ended, the phone rang. Shannon said Molly, our youngest granddaughter, wanted to come over to take Grandpa for a ride. They drove for about an hour, and then she took him home with her. I thought this was pretty amazing for a sixteen-year-old. About an hour later, Molly brought him home, because Gordon told her that he really thought he should get home to check on me.

In the late afternoon, he seemed a little better, at least quieter. He slept through his favorite TV show *Walker, Texas Ranger*, and although I woke him a couple of times, each time he went right back to sleep. He had had a very busy day and was exhausted … and that's a good thing!

9

Stories That Will Make You Cry

In 1997, we celebrated our fiftieth wedding anniversary. We had a group of one hundred-fifty people—friends and family from all over the country—for a sit-down dinner at the church. It was a wonderful evening, and Gordon recognized everyone but could not always put a name with the face. The light in his eyes indicated his recognition; our friends were pleased, and so was I.

A couple of days after the anniversary celebration, we were in the car running some errands. I could see out of the corner of my eye that he was studying me very carefully.

Finally, he leaned over and asked, "What is your name?"

"Jean," I answered.

"Oh yes," he said, "Jean Mack Pitzer."

About six months later, we were going to Oklahoma for my high school reunion. My sister Lucille was with us, and Gordon sat in the back seat. Lucille had brought a book on tape, Tom Brokaw's *The Greatest Generation*. I thought Gordon would enjoy it, because we both lived through the Depression, and he was very proud of the time he served in World War II. As we drove along, we listened to stories about the war.

After several minutes, Gordon leaned forward and asked, "Are we going to be bombed?"

I assured him we were not and turned off the tape. That was one time my idea did not work.

One morning several months later, we were walking across the parking lot on our way to church. Gordon was shuffling his feet. The noise was irritating to me, and I asked him, in not such a nice way, to pick up his feet. To this day, I can still see the hurt in his eyes. That was the last time I ever criticized him for anything. I was so ashamed of myself for being impatient. I have often said that I am the most impatient person in the world. But I do believe that when we ask, God has a way of changing us. People sometimes told me that they admired the way I handled Gordon and how patient I was with him. I always told them that it was a learned art. I certainly was not born that way. It isn't easy, but I urge every caregiver to be calm and patient.

For the first three years, there were days that were truly normal. We were able to discuss family matters. He was able to read the sports page and watch ball games on TV. I had always teased Gordon by saying that he would watch anything on TV as long as it involved at least two people and a ball.

Growing up, he had played basketball and football until he broke his arm at the age of eight. He only grew to be five foot seven, but he loved basketball and played it in high school and in college.

One of the saddest moments for me was when I visited him one day at the assisted-living home and there was a basketball tournament on TV, but he was not watching it. He was sitting just six feet away from the television. I said something about the game, and I got no response at all. He had lost one of the greatest loves of his life.

We had appointments with the neurologist every other month. Each time we went, he gave Gordon a battery of tests, with the same questions each month: "What year is this? What month? What day? What state do you live in? What town? What county? Where are you right now? In what year were you born? How old are you? Spell 'world' backward. Start at one hundred, subtract seven each time, and go as far as you can."

One day, the first question Gordon attempted to answer was his birthday, and he got it right. After that, his answers were not so accurate.

"Year born?"

"1888." (He was born in 1924.)

"How old are you?"

"Thirty-nine or forty-nine; I forget." (He was seventy-four.)

When the doctor asked who was president, Gordon couldn't remember Clinton's name. The doctor then asked what the president had done.

Gordon answered, "He did some stuff he shouldn't have done."

This was one of the brief moments of clarity that becomes treasured. After that day, though, the doctor stopped asking questions. It was unbelievable how fast Gordon's condition deteriorated. I wondered if it might taper off or even reverse …

Hope does spring eternal.

10

Stories to Amuse You

One night in the summer of 1998, I was getting the trash ready to take to the curb for pickup the next day. I had just taken the plastic liner out of the waste basket in the kitchen when the phone rang. I answered on the kitchen phone, and while I was talking, I heard a funny noise. When I looked around, I saw that Gordon had dropped his pants and was sitting on the trashcan attempting to urinate. I quickly ended the phone conversation and asked him if he needed to go to the bathroom.

His answer was, "I think I just did."

Later that same evening, I was again on the phone in the kitchen and saw Gordon with a full gallon of milk. He was pouring it onto the cabinet. I asked him if he wanted a glass of milk, and he nodded yes. As I grabbed a glass, I told him that we needed to put a glass under the mouth of the jug, to catch the milk that he was pouring. It didn't register at all. There are times when, if you don't laugh (or at least smile), you will find yourself crying.

As I have stated, I sing in the choir at church. One night, when Gordon had gotten to the point where I didn't feel comfortable leaving him home alone, I took him with me to choir practice. A friend told her husband about it when she got home and then called to say that her husband would come over every Thursday night to stay with Gordon while she and I went to choir practice. One night, while her husband was there, Gordon left the room, and our friend thought he had gone to the bathroom. He waited a couple of minutes before checking to see what was going on. Gordon had brought the garden hose (with the water running) into the living room and was watering the hardwood floor. The friend quickly grabbed the hose and asked Gordon to go to the den and stay there. He then proceeded to mop up the water.

When he returned to the den, Gordon was still sitting in his chair. He looked up and said, "You're not my boss."

Thank goodness the friend did not take this personally, and our Thursday night ritual continued.

Once, when John was home for a visit, he was sitting on the couch and Gordon and I were in our recliners. Gordon had his back to John and was trying to tell me something, but it was totally incoherent.

I just kept smiling and saying, "Oh really? I didn't know that. Okay … Really?"

Finally, John mouthed to me, "What is he saying?"

I shook my head and mouthed back to him, "I haven't a clue."

John was amused, because he had thought, by the way I was answering, that I had understood what his dad was saying.

One night, our friends arrived so that she and I could go to choir practice. I had gone to the bedroom to get my jacket, when the phone rang. I picked up the phone in the bedroom, but before I could answer, I heard Gordon saying, "Hello? Hello?"

His voice was not coming through the phone but from down the hall. I couldn't figure it out until I finished the short conversation and went into the den. He had picked up a paper cup and was holding it to his ear, saying, "Hello?"

11

Once in a While,
We Get It Right

Another important event was our trip to Kansas in May 2000. Gordon was to celebrate his fiftieth reunion at Sterling College. That is a good seven-hour drive, and I could find all kinds of reasons not to make the trip. However, none of them measured up to the reasons I *should* take him, and driving would actually be easier than flying, because there was no direct flight.

I called the girl in charge of the reunion reservations and told her that I wanted to bring Gordon but was afraid that at the last minute he might not feel like going. She urged me to bring him if at all possible and said she fully understood the situation. There would be a place for us, but if we needed to cancel at the last minute not to worry. I drove the trip in two days so neither of us would be too tired.

Everyone was so happy to see Gordon. His eyes lit up when he recognized someone. But things went downhill very fast as they continued to visit. He was so happy to be back in Sterling, but he could not express in words how happy he was. We all saw it through his eyes and his big smile, though! I will always be grateful for the inner voice that told me to make this trip.

By that summer I realized I must start looking for an assisted-living home. Gordon's condition was going downhill very rapidly. There was never any coherent conversation, and he was unable to dress himself. I could still handle these things, but if he continued on the downward spiral, I knew I probably would not be able to go it alone. One possibility was in-home care, but I couldn't be sure it would work.

I was told that I would have to undergo major surgery in September, and I would not be able to lift more than twenty pounds for two months after the surgery. I was pulling Gordon out of a chair or out of bed many times a day, as he had no strength left in his legs. I knew I couldn't continue to physically care for him.

I had heard about a new facility in town that was specifically for Alzheimer's patients. This assisted-living facility had a sliding scale in order to fill up the rooms. I knew I could not afford full price, and getting Medicaid help was very difficult. I visited the new facility and found it to be beautiful, clean, and comfortable, and the staff seemed very nice.

During that same week, I was informed that my surgery would be in November instead of September because of a conflict in the doctor's schedule. At that point I didn't know whether to get Gordon into assisted living then or to wait until November.

The following Sunday, I invited the choir director and another friend to have lunch with us after church. When Gordon finished eating, he left the table, and I thought he had gone into the den. A few minutes later, the doorbell rang. It was our next-door neighbor holding Gordon by the hand.

He said, "Jean, it's too hot out here for Gordon."

It was 109 degrees. That was the first time he had wandered off with my being unaware that he had left the house.

During church that morning, I had done nothing but pray for God to give me a sign as to when to get Gordon into assisted living. After the neighbor brought him home, I gave thanks to God for this sign. How could I have been so careless about where he was? He could have been in the heat long enough to have a heat stroke. He could have wandered out into a very busy street near our home. I could not believe this had happened.

By Friday, my kids and I got him moved into the assisted-living home. He seemed fairly content, until I was ready to leave after a visit. He would follow me down the hall, wanting to go home with me. I would stop and tell him I couldn't take him home because I had to have surgery. Although that seemed to suffice, the heartache I felt after putting him in the home was terribly difficult to handle.

I had just put my husband of fifty-three years in a home for strangers to take care of him. I had done it two months earlier than necessary. I had a hard time justifying that. My faith, my family, and my friends helped me through this crushing period in our journey.

After my successful surgery, I was telling a friend about my dilemma and how the Lord had worked things out.

Her answer was, "Jean, the Lord didn't work out the timing for Gordon; it was for you. The last several months you have looked so tired, and that is no way to go in for major surgery."

This made me realize that the timing was beneficial not only to Gordon but to me as well.

One day, soon after Gordon had entered the assisted-living facility, I went to the hospital to visit a friend who had recently been diagnosed with Alzheimer's. He was staring at the ceiling and yelling very loudly. A family member had turned a radio on and had the music terribly loud, because the patient supposedly loved music. I tried to talk to the patient, but I couldn't. Finally, I asked someone to turn the music down.

I held the man's hand and talked in a very low, soothing voice to him for a few minutes. He became very calm and soon went to sleep. The family was trying, to the best of their ability, to please him with the music, but it was having the opposite effect on him. I had learned from my experience how important it is for the family or caregiver to try new ideas to calm an Alzheimer's patient. If one thing doesn't work, try something else.

12

Looking for a Nursing Home

I truly thought Gordon would be in the assisted-living facility for three or four years. At the end of nine months, I was told that they could no longer keep him, because his condition had deteriorated so badly. The assisted living did not have twenty-four-hour nursing care, and the doctor had determined that Gordon needed constant care.

In the spring of 2001, after falling and hitting his head, Gordon was admitted to the hospital for tests. Thankfully, he had no serious head injury, but there was a concern about his food intake. Doctors tested his ability to swallow. Forgetting how to swallow is common in Alzheimer's patients. They found he still remembered how to swallow, but he had forgotten how to chew. He could no longer have solid food; everything had to be pureed.

While he was in the hospital, his roommate and I were talking one day while a nurse attended to Gordon. The man told me that I was amazing.

"Why in the world would you say something like that?" I asked.

He explained that when my husband first came in, his own family tried to talk to him, but they couldn't understand anything he said. Apparently this man thought I could understand everything Gordon said and that I was actually carrying on a conversation with him. I laughed to myself and explained to him that I really did not understand anything he said. All I knew was that he was evidently trying to tell me something, and my answering him calmed him down.

The doctor said I should let the social worker at the hospital find a nursing home, because, as he said, "She could open doors that I could not even find." I consulted her; she tried; but kept striking out.

One morning, she reported all of the places that she had tried, and they were all full.

I became very angry and said out loud, "What am I going to do? How can this be happening? He can't stay in the hospital, and the assisted living will not let me take him back there."

Suddenly, a peace came over me, and I calmed down and said, "I will do what I have done from the start of this nightmare. I will rely completely on my faith."

The very next morning when I got to the hospital, the social worker came running down the hall when she saw me.

"Mrs. Pitzer, I found one!"

By the next day, we had Gordon moved into a nursing home with a unit for Alzheimer's patients.

This was when I actually applied for Medicaid. I had talked to them much earlier but was told that I could not apply until Gordon was actually in the nursing home.

I did get the information at that time that his $40,000 in life insurance was twice as much as was allowed. The social worker informed me that I would have to cash in half that amount in order to be considered for Medicaid.

I did as I was told. As I could not keep the money, I used it to finish paying for his pre-paid burial policy and to pay off our few debts. I used some of the money to get the house in a more maintenance-free condition. Our home is brick, so I had siding put on the eaves to eliminate the need for repainting. We were also in need of a new refrigerator, so I bought and paid for that. Unlike Gordon, I do not enjoy yard work, so I had a sprinkler system installed.

Both Gordon and I had worked for years. He was with 3M for twenty-three years, and I had been with the University of Texas Southwestern Medical School in Dallas for fourteen years. Before that, I had worked as a church secretary for nine years and as a school secretary for eight years. We had very good benefits; however, none of the benefits covered long-term care.

Medicaid allows patients one home and one car but no CDs, 401Ks, or bonds. One can have a savings account if there is no more than $1,000 in it. I had to send Medicaid a copy of my bank statements, copies of insurance policies, and savings account reports for the prior three months. They make it very difficult for middle-class families to receive help.

I then had to get a Miller's Trust form from an attorney. This is an agreement between the power of attorney (me, in this case), the bank, and Medicaid to set up a separate account for the patient. Nothing goes into this account but the patient's retirement check or paycheck, as the circumstance might be. Subsequently, I wrote a check to the nursing home for the same amount each month. Gordon's retirement check was a mere pittance compared to the monthly bill at the nursing home. But they agreed to do this, thinking I would be approved by Medicaid and then Medicaid would pay the difference.

I also obtained a durable power of attorney for health issues and a power of attorney for business purposes, as well as a DNR (do not resuscitate). I learned that a copy of this needs to be filed with the nursing home, the hospital, and the doctor's office. All these things should be taken care of *before* they are needed, because when it is time for them, it may be too late to get them.

Medicaid never did approve us. I had a tax shelter annuity I had bought when I was at the medical school. I had money automatically taken out of my check each month to go to this fund. When I reached the age of 70½, I had to start taking the money out. Medicaid could not understand (or refused to understand) that I had no choice about cashing this in. Metropolitan, the life insurance company through which I had the tax shelter annuity, even sent them a letter stating that the fund was irrevocable. It could not be cashed in, but that did not get us approved for Medicaid. A year and a half after Gordon's death, I was still making monthly payments for his care. As I already stated, they make it very difficult for the middle class.

13

The Last Few Days

In early September 2001, when Gordon had been in the nursing home for about two months, he had a bad fall. He was taken to the hospital to have a gash on his head sewn up. No one saw him fall, and they never found out what he had hit. By this time he did not know me, nor did he know anyone else. But still, he surely hurt when he fell and struck his head; I could do nothing but pray that the Lord would take him home quickly and not let him suffer.

Three months after he went into the nursing home, he was taken to the hospital again. This time he was comatose. He had developed a bad bladder infection, which was due in part to the fact that he had forgotten how to swallow and was not getting enough fluids. He was checked into the hospital and put on antibiotics. After being there for four days, I was talking to the nurse and said something about him being there until the antibiotics cleared up the infection.

She said, "Mrs. Pitzer, antibiotics will not fix what is wrong with your husband."

Stunned, I thanked her for being so forthcoming about Gordon's condition. After praying about it, I contacted the doctor and had him take Gordon off the medication.

Before leaving the hospital, we signed up for hospice care. What a blessing this organization is—so caring and loving. They checked on Gordon at least three times a day, and the chaplain was available any time I needed him.

We took Gordon back to the nursing home on Thursday, September 13, 2001, two days after 9/11. I was so shocked and angry over what had happened to our country and all of the lives that had been lost. It was as though the whole world was falling apart and I was trying desperately to hold on. My emotions were torn, and the tears would not stop.

On the next Monday, the doctor informed us that Gordon probably had twenty-four hours to live. On Tuesday he gave him "twenty-four to forty-eight hours" to live. On Wednesday, I told him that one of our sons lived out of state and would be in that night at 7:40. He asked me to call and see if he could get an earlier flight.

"I want him here before his father dies," the doctor said softly.

This allowed our entire family to be present for Gordon's death. He lived another thirty-six hours. He had such a strong heart; if he had not had Alzheimer's or some other disease, I think he would have lived to be one hundred years old.

I had talked to a doctor at the nursing home about Gordon being an organ donor. I was informed that they do not take organs from Alzheimer's patients for fear of giving the recipient the disease. Neither could we donate his cornea, as they do not take these from persons over the age of sixty-five.

A year after Gordon's death, I heard a doctor give a talk on the importance of organ donations. His opinion contradicted our experience. He said there were only two criteria for not using the organs from a patient: if the patient was HIV positive or had metastatic cancer. He also said that there is no age limit. He knew of successful transplants from a patient ninety-two years old.

When it was time for questions, I asked about Alzheimer's. He then reiterated his previous statement, so I told him my story about trying to donate. He told me we were given very bad information. I felt sick to my stomach to think that someone could have used Gordon's organs to have a new life—especially his strong heart.

I wrote to the medical director of the nursing home and told her about my new information. I simply asked that they educate their staff so this does not happen again. So many lives can be saved if healthy organs are not buried!

In the days after Gordon's death, the boys and I made funeral arrangements and plans for a memorial service. We had the burial on Monday morning and a memorial service that night. John presided and preached his father's funeral, and Jim gave a talk. I was so proud of them both.

I thought I was prepared for the end, but I was not. We had bought our cemetery lots several years ago, had prepaid funeral expenses, and I had written the obituary several months before needing it. In fact, I had written both Gordon's and my own and then attached a picture to each of them to be used in the newspaper. These are things that the kids would have struggled with, so I decided to make it as easy as possible. I also made a list of songs and scriptures I would like used in the memorial services.

At the top of the obituaries I wrote a note to the boys: "This is a starting place; feel free to change it any way you wish." Then I filed them and told the boys and Shannon where to find them.

I had been living alone for a year, but actually I had been alone for about five years. Gordon had left me mentally long before he went to the assisted-living facility. I thought I had adjusted to the empty house, but it was different now. Every time I saw something of Gordon's, every time I saw his picture, every time he was mentioned, it made me realize, again, that he was not coming home.

In time, I knew I must get involved in outside activities again and not dwell on the past. I was so glad I had not given up my volunteer work. I started taking oil painting classes again and joined Bible Study Fellowship, better known as BSF. I also continue with my Wednesday evening dinner group.

I would urge anyone who has been through this to get out of the house and make a new life. Make new friends, learn a new language, tutor, or volunteer. There are so many children struggling in school, and a tutor could make such a difference in their lives. Travel, and ask a friend to go with you. It helps to keep active and busy. Giving back to the world was Gordon's way of living. I honor his memory by continuing to honor this concept.

As most of us know, there is no known cure for Alzheimer's at this time, but there have been many articles written on how we can help to protect ourselves. Even though we cannot prove anything, it certainly makes sense that we should eat healthfully and try to take care of our bodies. We know the disease is not contagious but genetics is recognized as a factor in Alzheimer's. The more we do to maintain a healthy lifestyle the more we help ourselves in the long run.

According to nutritional experts, we must make changes in our diets. It might be too late for your loved one who is living with Alzheimer's, but it is not too late for you and your children, grandchildren, and friends.

Researchers at the USDA Human Nutrition Research Center on Aging at Tufts University have found in studies that foods containing high levels of antioxidants show great potential in fighting off multiple diseases, including Alzheimer's.

In general, dark-skinned fruits and vegetables have the highest levels of naturally occurring antioxidants. Such fruits include blueberries, blackberries, strawberries, raspberries, plums, oranges, cherries, and red grapes. Vegetables with high antioxidant levels include kale, spinach, brussell sprouts, alfalfa sprouts, broccoli, beets, red bell pepper, and eggplant.

In addition to fruits and vegetables, cold-water fish contain beneficial omega-3 fatty acids, which are also considered good brain food. Halibut, mackerel, salmon, trout, and tuna are examples of these fish.

This same study shows the importance of lifestyle changes that can help reduce your risk of Alzheimer's disease or other dementia. Staying mentally active, remaining socially involved, and staying physically active are extremely important as you attempt to find ways to lower your risk of Alzheimer's.[1]

The Alzheimer's Association has also listed ten warning signs of Alzheimer's Disease. The signs are:

1. *Memory loss.* Forgetting recently learned information is one of the most common early signs of dementia. A person begins to forget more often and is unable to recall the information later. What is normal? Forgetting names or appointments occasionally.

2. *Difficulty performing familiar tasks.* People with dementia often find it hard to plan or complete everyday tasks. Individuals may lose track of the steps involved in preparing a meal, placing a telephone call, or playing a game. What is normal? Occasionally forgetting why you came into a room or what you planned to say.

3. *Problems with language.* People with Alzheimer's disease often forget simple words or substitute them with unusual words, making their speech or writing hard to understand. They may be unable to find the toothbrush, for example, and instead ask

---

1.   USDA Human Nutrition Research Center on Aging at Tufts University

for "that thing for my mouth." What is normal? Sometimes having trouble finding the right word.

4. *Disorientation of time and place.* People with Alzheimer's disease can become lost in their own neighborhood, forget where they are and how they got there, and may not know how to get back home. What is normal? Forgetting the day of the week or where you were going.

5. *Poor or decreased judgment.* Those with Alzheimer's may dress inappropriately, wearing several layers on a warm day or little clothing in the cold. What is normal? Making a questionable or debatable decision from time to time.

6. *Problems with abstract thinking.* Someone with Alzheimer's disease may have unusual difficulty performing complex mental tasks, like forgetting what numbers are for and how they should be used. What is normal? Finding it challenging to balance a checkbook.

7. *Misplacing things.* A person with Alzheimer's disease may put things in unusual places: an iron in the freezer or a wristwatch in the sugar bowl. What is normal? Misplacing keys or a wallet temporarily.

8. *Changes in mood or behavior.* Someone with Alzheimer's disease may show rapid mood swings—from calm to tears to anger—for no apparent reason. What is normal? Occasionally feeling sad or moody.

9. *Changes in personality.* The personalities of people with dementia can change dramatically. They may become extremely confused, suspicious, fearful, or dependent on a family member.

What is normal? People's personalities do change somewhat with age.

10. *Loss of initiative.* A person with Alzheimer's disease may become very passive, sitting in front of the TV for hours, sleeping more than normal, or not wanting to participate in usual activities. What is normal? Sometimes feeling weary of work or social obligations.[2]

---

2.   Published in the Fort Worth Star Telegram August 16, 2006

14

Helpful Suggestions

If you suspect that a loved one has early signs of Alzheimer's ...

1. *Seek help immediately.* It is very easy to ignore what is right in front of you. There might even be times of complete denial, but becoming proactive instead of reactive really is the way to go. Ask your friends to recommend a good neurologist in your area. Go online and source out all the valid information you can find. Remember, knowledge is a most powerful tool.

2. *Let the patient talk or even ramble.* Don't feel bad if you can't understand him or her; one thing I learned early was never to disagree with something Gordon said. If I did, he became extremely agitated. I just left it alone, regardless of how wild or weird; I did not correct him. If anyone was around, they understood. After it became impossible to understand what he was saying, I would listen and then say, "Really?" or "I didn't know that," or some other phrase that came to mind.

3. *Make nutritional changes.* Eat less fat and more fruits and vegetables. The Alzheimer's Association suggests that if you have Alzheimer's in your family, you should eat a half-cup of blueberries a day.

4. *Try taking a drive.* I found this to be helpful and calming for the patient.

5. *Allow them to dress themselves for as long as possible.* Once you start doing everything for the patient they will not try to help themselves and the downhill slide goes faster.

6. *Trust your instincts.* If you learn to rely on your inner voice, it will save you a great deal of second-guessing. If you know deep down that something is wrong, seek help. If you know you need a break, find help. If you know you don't have all of the answers, just ask.

7. *When planning something special …* Do not tell the patient about an upcoming event until it is time to get ready. This will save you a great deal of frustration.

8. *Come up with inventive ways to give meds.* For example, crush the pills, use a spoon to get the meds further into the mouth and then give them water to swallow the meds.

FRIENDS OF CAREGIVERS, PLEASE INSIST ON HELPING. The caregiver may very well resist your help, because it is easy to get into the mind-set of "I can do it all." Thank goodness I had very persistent friends who insisted on helping, taking me out to dinner, and finding someone to sit with Gordon. If you know a caregiver, I *urge* you to call them and offer them your time.

CAREGIVERS, ACCEPT HELP THAT IS OFFERED TO YOU.

15

Conclusion

In looking back over the last seventy-nine years, it is easy to see where my life has been filled with great joy and happiness. There certainly have been times of struggle, but I must say that I am very blessed with a wonderful and loving family, caring friends, and a faith that allows me to face each day knowing that all will be well. One of my greatest blessings was walking hand in hand with my husband for over fifty years. Only God could have brought together a young man from Pennsylvania and a young woman from Oklahoma, to have us meet in Kansas during our college years.

So, this book has simply been a reflection of part of that fifty-year journey. When I reflect on these almost six years since Gordon passed away, I can only wonder in amazement at everything I have learned. It is my hope, therefore, that you have not only learned something about Alzheimer's disease by reading this book but also discovered new things about yourself. Take that new knowledge and make good things happen. Help a caregiver, volunteer—become a believer in the power of people and the common good.

I also urge you to be generous in making a contribution to Alzheimer's research. I have made that commitment, and I hope you will as well. Just imagine if everyone affected by this disease made a monthly donation. Great things would happen!

If you would like more information, please contact your local Alzheimer's Association. If your town does not have one, you can locate the association on the World Wide Web at www.alzheimers.org, or you can write the national research headquarters. The address is given below.

Alzheimer's Disease Research
1230 York Avenue
New York, NY 10021

You Too Can Survive

Gordon Pitzer was diagnosed with Alzheimer's disease in 1995. Six year later, he was gone.

Compiled by his wife, Jean Pitzer, *You Too Can Survive* is the moving story of his Alzheimer's experience. More than that, it chronicles Jean's experience as Gordon's caregiver. It highlights her emotional hills and valleys and expands upon what she has learned during her caregiver process.

Each of the fourteen chapters gives accounts of their day-to-day Alzheimer-afflicted world.

You Too Can Survive is important reading for anyone currently experiencing Alzheimer's in their own life.

978-0-595-41068-2
0-595-41068-5

Printed in the United States
96609LV00008B/251/A